2018

Comfrey root the miracle plant

WRITTEN BY

MARIA D. TALTON

TABLE OF CONTENTS

What Is Comfrey?

Comfrey is a bush that develops in parts of Europe, Asia, and North America. It can grow up to 5 feet tall. It produces groups of purple, blue, and white blooms, and it's acclaimed for its long, thin leaves and dark cleaned roots.

In herbal medicine, we have utilized the roots and leaves of Comfrey, a quickly developing, extensive plant that structures a 'rosette' of spear molded leaves (up to 30cms long) that set up a tall blooming stem up to 1.5 meters high. Comfrey leaves have numerous restorative properties; they are unpleasant finished and canvassed in short solid hairs. The roots are additionally extremely well known in home grown medication, they are short, thick, and many-extended and they have a dark surface with a white, chewy, somewhat sweet inside.

The root and leaves of the comfrey plant have been utilized as a part of conventional medication in numerous parts of the world. In Japan, the plant has been gathered and utilized as a customary treatment for more than 2,000 years. It was initially called "knit bone" and individuals utilized it to treat:

- muscle sprains
- wounds
- consumes
- joint aggravation

Europeans have additionally utilized comfrey to treat incendiary conditions, for example, joint pain and gout. Some conventional healers have additionally utilized it to treat looseness of the bowels and other stomach afflictions.

The underlying foundations of leaves of the comfrey plant contain concoction substances called allantoin and rosmarinic corrosive. Allantoin supports the development of new skin cells, while rosmarinic corrosive eases agony and irritation. Concentrates are as yet produced using the roots and leaves and transformed into balms, creams, or treatments. These arrangements commonly have a comfrey substance of 5 to 20 percent.

While comfrey is outstanding for its medical advantages, it likewise represents a few dangers. It contains aggravates that can hurt your liver. It might likewise be cancer-causing. Therefore, numerous nations have restricted the offer of oral comfrey arrangements. Numerous specialists likewise prompt against utilizing topical comfrey on open injuries.

Be that as it may, comfrey might be adequate for here and now use on your skin and shut injuries. You can buy topical comfrey arrangements from numerous wellbeing stores. Converse with your specialist before utilizing them to take in more about the potential advantages and dangers.

History

Comfrey has been developed since around 400 BC as a recuperating herb. The word comfrey, got from the Latin word for "become together", mirrors the early employments of this plant. Greeks and Romans utilized comfrey to stop overwhelming dying, treat bronchial issues, and recuperate wounds and broken bones. Poultices were made for outside injuries and tea was devoured for interior diseases.

Comfrey (Symphytum spp.) is local to Europe and Asia. In spite of the fact that comfrey has been utilized as a sustenance edit, and as a scrounge trim, in the previous 20 years logical investigations detailed that comfrey might be cancer-causing, since it seemed to cause liver harm and malignant tumors in rats. Comfrey-pepsin cases, which are sold as a stomach related guide in natural and wellbeing nourishment stores in the USA, have been broke down and found to contain pyrrolizidine alkaloids. These alkaloids cause liver harm in individuals and are a potential cancer-causing agent. Huxtable et al. (1986) refered to instances of hepatic veno-occlusive malady that were delivered by utilizing these containers. These reports have briefly confined improvement of comfrey as a sustenance edit.

Three plant species in the family Symphytum are important to the product known as comfrey. Wild or regular comfrey, Symphytum officinale L., is local to England and stretches out all through the vast majority of Europe into Central Asia and Western Siberia. Thorny or harsh comfrey [S. asperum Lepechin (S. asperrimum Donn)], named for its bristly or bushy leaves, was conveyed to Britain from Russia around 1800. Quaker, Russian, or blue comfrey [S. × uplandicum Nyman (S. peregrinum Lebed.)] started as a characteristic half and half of S. officinale L. what's more, S. asperum Lepechin. This cross breed was called Russian or

Caucasian comfrey in reference to its nation of source. Cuttings of this cross breed were transported to Canada in 1954 and it was named Quaker comfrey, after the religion of Henry Doubleday, the British analyst in charge of advancing comfrey as a sustenance and rummage. The larger part of comfrey developed in the United States can be followed to this presentation.

Verifiably, cultivator's utilized oral and topical cures containing comfrey root to advance the recuperating of bones, gaining the herb the Latin name Symphytum, signifying "drawing together," and the basic names knit bone and boneset. Cultivator's likewise utilized creams produced using comfrey root to apply topically to wounds, sprains or strains, wounds and varicose veins, says the University of Pittsburgh Medical Center. Individuals additionally took the root orally to treat lung issues, stomach ulcers and other gastrointestinal issues, and an eyewash produced using comfrey was utilized to treat eye issues and disturbances, takes note of the University of Michigan Health System.

As a portion of its different names recommend, (knit bone, boneset) Comfrey has been prized since antiquated circumstances for its capacity to help recuperate broken bones and harmed tissues. In present day times, it has been found this is in any event to some degree because of a substance in Comfrey called 'allantoin' that can quicken cell 'mitosis', which means it speeds the procedure of new tissue development.

Comfrey has been verifiably utilized for all way of wounds and mischances including however not constrained to broken bones. It has a similarly solid notoriety for assisting with outside injuries that are inadequately recuperating.

Comfrey has been utilized for ulceration anyplace along the gastrointestinal tract, for seeping from the stomach, throat, inside, bladder and lungs. Comfrey used to be utilized widely for tuberculosis and disturbing dry lung dissensions as a rule.

Location of comfrey

Comfrey is an individual from the Boraginaceae family whose major observable attributes incorporate somewhat blue blossoms and bristly hairs and is of the class Symphytum. There are three plant species in the family Symphytum that are applicable to the product known as Comfrey. Wild, or basic Comfrey (Symphytum officinale) is local to England and reaches out all through the majority of Europe into Central Asia and Western Siberia. Thorny or harsh Comfrey (Symphytum asperrimum), named for its bristly leaves, was conveyed to England from Russia around 1800. Quaker, Russian, or blue Comfrey started as a characteristic half breed of S. officinale and S. asperrimum. This mixture was called Caucasian or Russian comfrey in reference to its nation of starting point. Cuttings of this cross breed were transported to Canada in 1954 and it was named Quaker Comfrey after the religion of Henry Doubleday, the British analyst in charge of advancing Comfrey as a nourishment and scavenge plant. The greater part of Comfrey developed monetarily in the United States seems to originate from these same plants delivered to Canada and got from the British Bocking Mixture (where they were developed is Bocking, England), which is a blend of a few clones that vary somewhat in plant life and general natural structure.

The Comfrey plant is a low, thick bush whose stems can achieve three to five feet in tallness. Being a lasting herb, it bites the dust back in the winter. The leaves are coarse and shaggy; fastening and substitute (without stipules) on the stem and their edge is whole. The measure of the leaves ranges from five to twelve inches winding up continuously littler toward the highest point of the plant. The blooms are purplish, white or light yellow and each single one is tubular formed and about a half inch long. They arrive in a cyme (group of 15-20 blossoms for each peduncle) and are scorpioid in their development design. The calyx comprises of five sepals, the corolla is five lobed and the blossom has five anthers. The nutlet is profoundly installed in the calyx of each blossom. The roots are short, thick and tuberous and the whole root framework is sweeping and develops as profound as eight feet into the ground.

The plant requires profound, however not really great, soil for development. Efficiency isn't exceptionally touchy to soil pH, however most elevated yields happen on soils with a pH of 6.0 to 7.0. The perfect planting times are in the spring and Comfrey is best spread by division, not seed. It delivers its most noteworthy yields in full daylight and under cooler conditions, however, it is dry season safe because of its broad root framework. It favors clammy, ripe soil, however is versatile to numerous sorts of soil. Comfrey plantings are known to last uncertainly (over twenty years) if soil ripeness and legitimate weed control are kept up and are best planted three to four feet separated from each other. Comfrey is a high-protein scavenge that acquires the greater part of its nitrogen from the dirt; accordingly, this supplement must be added to the dirt through treating the soil and preparation. It drives its underlying foundations profound into the dirt, raising calcium, phosphorus and potash, and in addition numerous follow components.

Sicknesses are not a difficult issue here in the United States. In England, Comfrey rust organism (Melampsorella symphyti) overwinters in the roots and diminishes the measure of old plantings gathered, however this malady has not spread to the U.S. because of plant isolate directions on the importation of plants or roots. There haven't been any creepy crawly issues announced in the U.S. identified with Comfrey.

Comfrey is likewise prescribed as a manure in the garden since its carbon to nitrogen proportion is around 14 to 1. At the point when compost is made we are utilizing microbes to bring down the extent of carbon to nitrogen mixes so as to create warm. It is compost which makes a garden into a flourishing spot, as well, since it makes the minerals and supplements that plants require promptly accessible to them. The normal proportion of carbon to nitrogen is 10 to 1. Along these lines, Comfrey is about manure before it goes on the store! The accompanying is a formula for Comfrey compost:

"Pick a decent measured bunch of clears out. Place them in a compartment with enough water to cover the clears out. Cover and let this cook for a month in cool climate or 2 weeks in sweltering climate. At that point crush the leaves to remove however much squeeze as could reasonably be expected. Strain and use at a rate of 1/some comfrey juice to one gallon of water. Use as a foliar feed and soil douse around the plants....the smell while it is cooking is solid!"

Comfrey used for skin regeneration

When you consider that our skin is the biggest organ of our bodies, it's reasonable that there are such huge numbers of solutions for managing topical inconveniences. Scratches, cuts, nibbles, consumes, rashes and wounds are among the huge number of conditions that can antagonistically influence skin. Also, for all intents and purposes every one of them, there's comfrey.

Local to Europe, comfrey is an expansive leafed garden plant whose well-known green leaves are secured with fluffy hairs. Otherwise called knit bone, knit back and ass– ear, the plant is supported by natural nursery workers for its dirt building properties, and adored by botanists for its skin-mending powers. The plant is high in protein, and develops plentifully. At the point when in sprout, comfrey has little white, pink or purple blooms. The plant's pretty appearance and strength make it a mainstream decorative.

Comfrey isn't new, and comfrey ointments, emollients and creams have been around for a considerable length of time. However a great many people still don't have the foggiest idea about this powerful skin-mending plant. In different arrangements, both Russian comfrey (Symphytum uplandicum) and normal comfrey (Symphytum officinale) are utilized. The name comfrey signifies "to become together," fitting for a plant used to mend wounds.

Comfrey ointments and other topical arrangements have for some time been utilized to recuperate wounds, skin ulcers and joint aggravation, and to assist breaks with knitting all the more rapidly. Comfrey arrangements are staples in Russian, European and North American herbology. In these, both the leaves and the foundations of the plant are utilized.

Normally comfrey is finely macerated and after that blended with a case, for example, beeswax, or a latent cream recipe. Comfrey can likewise be utilized in a shower by making an expansive pot of concentrated tea, adding to a shower, and absorbing the shower for some time. This improves and embellishes skin, and is relieving in instances of irritated and dry skin.

In the event that comfrey has a particularly strong skin-recuperating operator, it is allantoin, which can be discovered broadly in corrective arrangements, particularly those for delicate skin. It helps wound repair, quickens skin mending, and has mitigating action. Allantoin is the subject of numerous licenses, and is both gotten from comfrey and blended in research centers. Utilized in shampoos, toothpastes, healthy skin moisturizers, hostile to skin inflammation arrangements and lipstick, allantoin is a staple compound in the corrective business.

However different mixes in comfrey additionally exhibit benefits when connected to skin. Extra mixes including caffeic corrosive, chlorogenic corrosive and rosmarinic corrosive help to secure the lipid linings of skin cells, diminish aggravation, and show hostile to tumor movement. This may bolster the utilization of comfrey arrangements for different skin tumors.

In human clinical examinations, comfrey arrangements have performed well. In one examination, sufferers of intense lower leg sprains experienced more quick recuperation with the use of a comfrey-based cream. The readiness diminished swelling, lightened agony, and enhanced joint versatility. In another examination, comfrey cream indicated an incentive in decreasing lower back torment and enhancing osteoarthritis in the knee.

What's more, in yet another examination, the individuals who used a concentrated comfrey cream to treat skin scraped spots experienced more fast mending and recuperation than the individuals who did not.

Comfrey ointment, analgesic or cream is on my must-have list for an all-around loaded home pharmaceutical bureau. Most topical natural arrangements contain some comfrey, however some are more thought. I like the EuroPharma Traumaplant Comfrey Cream.

Since quite a while ago utilized, clinically tried, simple to develop, inexhaustible, shoddy and viable, comfrey merits its persisting spot in nature's pharmaceutical chest. Given its various advantages to the biggest human organ, comfrey is a decent solution for keep close by.

....

Comfrey as a remedy

Individuals still utilize comfrey as an elective solution for joint and muscle torment, and shut injuries. It's accessible at numerous wellbeing stores and drug stores as

- ointments
- creams
- other topical solutions
- salves that also contain other herbs, such as aloe and goldenseal

Wounds

Some clinical research underpins the claim that comfrey has wound-mending powers. For instance, an examination survey distributed in the diary Complementary Therapies in Medicine discovered some proof that comfrey can help recuperate scraped spot wounds. The creators take note of that topical uses of comfrey have all the earmarks of being protected, however more research is important to find out about the potential dangers and symptoms of utilizing comfrey on your skin and wounds.

Joint pain

As indicated by a similar research audit, comes about additionally proposed that comfrey can help treat osteoarthritis, and additionally a few wounds, for example, lower leg sprains. An investigation detailed in Phytotherapy Research additionally proposes that creams containing comfrey root can help assuage upper and lower back agony.

....

Medical use and safety

Extra uses of Comfrey leaf and root are no issue as far as potential poisonous quality and they work perfectly. I utilize a lot of Comfrey leaf and root in packs and creams for a man who has wounds or injuries that are not mending admirably.

In any case, the interior utilization of Comfrey must be attempted with awesome affectability and mind or not in any way. Comfrey can possibly hurt the liver. Comfrey has performed encourage little marvels in my training right up 'til the present time yet I utilize it infrequently and greatly precisely (doing successive blood tests in my center while the patient is utilizing it to search for trademark signs of liver pressure). I would guide any individual who isn't prepared in natural solution or who has experienced thorough examination into the logical writing on Comfrey basically to just not self-cure with this plant inside.

My musings on when the inward utilize is advocated are very much spoken to here by the immense English cultivator Thomas Bartram. He keeps in touch with 'Doubtlessly the utilization of the foundation of Symphytum officinale might be supported in the treatment of extreme bone ailments for which it has made a measure of progress before, for example, rickets, Paget's illness, broken bones and so forth its advantages exceeding dangers. Barely any other restorative plants recharge squandered bone cells with the speed of Comfrey'

Comfrey joins amazingly well with Calendula and Plantain to encourage recuperating and for some individuals it will be significantly smarter to utilize both of those awesome herbs for any inward 'injuries' and after that exclusive include the Comfrey if the treatment is to be utilized remotely. Comfrey can likewise work especially well with a little Licorice or Marshmallow pull for breaks, cuts and dry skin issues that are not mending admirably.

A 2004 twofold visually impaired investigation of 142 individuals experiencing lower leg sprains found that applying comfrey root extricate cream lessened mending time, torment and swelling throughout eight days, contrasted with fake treatment, says the University of Pittsburgh Medical Center. Another twofold visually impaired clinical preliminary distributed in 2009 found that comfrey root extricate salve treated intense back agony, as per the Memorial Sloan-Kettering Cancer Center. A three-week-long, twofold visually impaired investigation of 220 individuals distributed in 2006 likewise found that comfrey root extricate salve assuaged side effects identified with osteoarthritis of the knee, contrasted with fake treatment. A 2007 investigation of mice showed that comfrey root extricate had antiproliferative activities in hepatic malignancy cells. At long last, a 2007 twofold visually impaired investigation of 278 individuals with new skin scraped spots established that applying a 10-percent fixation comfrey cream expanded injury mending speed after only a few days. None of these investigations and clinical preliminaries demonstrate that comfrey root is protected and successful for treating any restorative condition, so make sure to counsel your doctor before utilizing comfrey cures.

The pyrrolizidine alkaloids contained in comfrey root can genuinely hurt your liver and might be cancer-causing. A few cases distributed in 1999 revealed that individuals created perilous liver issues or liver illness in the wake of taking comfrey root extricate cases or teas, says the University of Michigan Health System. Indeed, even here and now inward utilization of comfrey root concentrate can cause liver disappointment, notwithstanding prompting the requirement for a liver transplant. Actually, the U.S. Sustenance and Drug Administration requested that all supplements containing comfrey root be pulled from store retires because of the liver danger dangers. In spite of the fact that you're most in danger for liver harm when you take comfrey root cures orally, topical applications may likewise be risky in light of the fact that you can assimilate pyrrolizidine alkaloids through your skin. In this way, you shouldn't utilize comfrey removes before first chatting with a social insurance expert, or utilize separates containing in excess of 100 mcg of pyrrolizidine alkaloids in every day by day measurement. Additionally, don't utilize comfrey root extricate creams or treatments for longer than 10 back to back days or over a month and a half in a solitary year.

Cultivation

The Russian comfrey "Bocking 14" cultivar was created amid the 1950s by Lawrence D Hills, the organizer of the Henry Doubleday Research Association (the natural cultivating association itself named after the Quaker pioneer who initially brought Russian comfrey into Britain in the nineteenth century) following preliminaries at Bocking, close Braintree.

The comfrey bed ought to be all around arranged by weeding completely, and dressing with excrement if accessible. Counterbalances ought to be planted 0.6– 1 m (2 ft. 0 in– 3 ft. 3 in) separated with the developing focuses just underneath the surface, while root sections ought to be covered around 5 cm (2.0 in) profound. Keep the bed very much watered until the point when the youthful plants are built up. Comfrey ought not to be gathered in its first season as it needs to end up set up. Any blooming stems ought to be evacuated as these will debilitate the plant in its first year.

Comfrey is a quickly developing plant, delivering gigantic measures of leaf amid the developing season, and thus is nitrogen hungry. In spite of the fact that it is a tireless cultivator, it will profit by the expansion of creature fertilizer connected as a mulch, and can likewise be mulched with other nitrogen rich materials, for example, garden clippings. It is one of only a handful couple of plants that will endure the utilization of new pee weakened 50:50 with water, despite the fact that this ought not be routinely included as it might expand salt levels in the dirt and effectsly affect soil life, for example, worms. Develop comfrey plants can be collected up to four or five times each year. They are prepared for cutting when around 60 cm (24 in) high, and, contingent upon occasional conditions, this is typically in mid-Spring. Comfrey will quickly regrow, and will be prepared for additionally cutting around 5 weeks after the fact. It is said that the best time to cut comfrey is in the blink of an eye before blossoming, for this is the point at which it is at its most strong as far as the supplements that it offers. Comfrey can keep developing into mid-pre-winter, however it isn't fitting to keep taking cuttings after early harvest time so as to enable the plants to develop winter holds. After the developing season, leaving comfrey beds decrepit may convey higher yields in future harvests, as the plant develops vitality saves in its roots.

Comfrey ought to be collected by utilizing either shears, a sickle, or a grass shearer to trim the plant around 2 creeps over the ground, taking consideration taking care of it in light of the fact that the leaves and stems are canvassed in hairs that can bother the skin. It is prudent to wear gloves when taking care of comfrey. Regardless of being sterile, Bocking 14 Russian comfrey will relentlessly increment in measure. It is in this manner fitting to part it up like clockwork. It is anyway hard to expel comfrey once settled as it is profound establishing, and any parts left in the dirt will regrow. Rotovation can be fruitful, yet may take a few seasons. The most ideal approach to annihilate comfrey is to precisely uncover it, evacuating however much of the root as could be expected. This is best done in sweltering, dry summer climate, wherein the dry conditions will execute off any residual root stumps. Comfrey is for the most part inconvenience free once settled, albeit weaker or focused on plants can experience the ill effects of comfrey rust or buildup. Both are contagious sicknesses, despite the fact that they once in a while genuinely decrease plant development and therefore don't for the most part require control. Be that as it may, contaminated plants ought not to be utilized for proliferation purposes.

Benefits of Comfrey for skin, hair and health

Comfrey is known to be a skin-accommodating herb. As said previously, comfrey is rich in allantoin, a compound which comes stuffed with synthetics that guide in cell recovery and development and shields your skin from harm. On account of this property, comfrey offers various skincare advantages, for example,

1. Moisturization

Poultices and treatments produced using comfrey leaf oil help support and saturate your skin abandoning it delicate and supple. Being home grown in nature, this is ideal for those whose skin is touchy to synthetic compounds.

2. Skin Toning

Comfrey herbs have astringent properties, which helps draw the phones together with the goal that your skin seems tight and conditioned.

3. Expulsion of Blemishes

The allantoin contained in comfrey herb helps battle undesirable dull spots and flaws on your skin. The saturating properties of this plant will likewise encourage smooth out harsh and harmed skin and evacuate dead skin cells. Applying comfrey oil or treatments routinely will abandon you with faultless, flaw free skin.

4. Cures Skin Diseases and Conditions

The allantoin content in comfrey leaves and roots with their capacity to repair harmed cells and deliver new ones may help speed the mending of skin consumes, bug nibbles and rashes, skin ulcers, and bed injuries. It can cure different skin conditions like psoriasis, a condition where the skin winds up bothersome and red and has layered patches, and dermatitis, where patches of skin turn out to be unpleasant and excited, causing agonizing rankles. You can either decide to straightforwardly apply comfrey salve or a poultice produced using the smashed leaves of the herb or by drinking comfrey tea produced using comfrey root powder extricate.

Who doesn't need for a sound, radiant mane? Quit utilizing synthetic items that will just harm the state of your hair, you can show signs of improvement comes about by presenting comfrey in your hair mind schedule. This roots and the leaves of this herb is known to:

5. Control Hair Loss

Comfrey herbs contain plant proteins and are pressed with fundamental minerals, cancer prevention agents, and vitamin A. Applying comfrey oil straightforwardly into your scalp or drinking comfrey root tea can help turn around male pattern baldness.

6. Conditions Hair

Locally acquired shampoos and conditioners contain unfortunate sulfur aggravates that strip your hair of all its basic oils. Comfrey, then again, is a characteristic conditioner that can help tackle dry scalp issues, for example, dandruff, and furthermore conditions and sustains the hair to influence it to look glistening and sparkling.

7. Detangles Hair

Adhesive, a plant protein, contained in comfrey unwinds your hair and effortlessly detangles ties so you don't need to experience long periods of dissatisfaction after you venture out of the shower.

8. Treating Open Wounds and Diabetic Sores

Comfrey leaves can be squashed, squeezed, and connected as a wet glue specifically on open injuries and diabetic bruises. This can help stop germ develop that might be in charge of causing contaminations.

9. Recuperating Bruises and Bleeding

Comfrey leaves and roots are wealthy in tannins, a sort of intensify that astringently affects veins. The tannin is exclusively in charge of making comfrey herb so compelling in controlling dying. In this manner, applying a poultice made of comfrey root powder and leaf squeeze, or drinking tea made of comfrey root powder can enormously help in curing nosebleeds, seeping in skin wounds, and in lessening and speeding the mending of wounds.

10. Stomach related Aid

Comfrey tea has for some time been utilized as a powerful characteristic solution for alleviating the gastrointestinal tract to cure issues, for example, heartburn, indigestion, and acid reflux.

11. Repairing Bone Fractures

Applying comfrey oil to torn tendons or broken bones when it's unrealistic to put throws can help in advancing quick mending. The rosmarinic corrosive in comfrey helps in the recovery of new cells and can even remake torn and harmed muscles.

12. Curing Dental Problems

Comfrey pull powder is extraordinary for curing cavities and redrawing teeth, on account of the capacity of this herb to quicken teeth and tissue development.

You can utilize either dried or new or dried comfrey root. In case you're utilizing the dried root, rehydrate it first by delicately bubbling it for ten minutes. Mix in about a square inch of the rehydrated root with a few tablespoons of water to make a fluid and whirl this around in your mouth for around 20 minutes every day. Guarantee to flush your mouth with this fluid such that it achieves your gums and your teeth appropriately. Once you're done, spit it out.

13. Mitigating Pain and Inflammation

Old Greeks and Romans swung to the comfrey leaves to recuperate breaks. The calming properties of this herb make it extremely viable in recuperating torment rapidly. Drinking comfrey tea or applying a poultice straightforwardly to throbbing joints can likewise help cure rheumatoid joint inflammation and osteoarthritis.

14. Curing Diaper Rash in Babies

Salves and mellow poultices influenced utilizing comfrey to leaf concentrates can help assuage babies from diaper rash. This intense, yet mellow home grown mixture works tenderly on your infant's sensitive skin. It is, be that as it may, best to first test this treatment to perceive how your child's skin responds to it. Apply somewhat first to complete a little fix test. On the off chance that that piece of your child's skin doesn't hint at any disturbance, you can keep applying the treatment.

....

References

https://www.healthline.com/health/what-is-comfrey#risks

https://www.livestrong.com/article/360851-nutritional-value-of-licorice-root/

http://www.rjwhelan.co.nz/herbs%20A-Z/comfreyroot.html

http://www.herballegacy.com/ThesisLocation.html

https://en.wikipedia.org/wiki/Comfrey

https://hort.purdue.edu/newcrop/afcm/comfrey.html

http://www.foxnews.com/health/2013/09/18/comfrey-topical-rescue-from-skin-healing-plant.html https://www.curejoy.com/content/benefits-of-comfrey-for-skin-hair-and-health/

www.ingramcontent.com/pod-product-compliance
Lightning Source LLC
Chambersburg PA
CBHW051142250726
48655CB00007B/3191